Breathing & Life

Hyo Hun Kang

I. PROLOGUE

As a child, I was always interested in the martial arts. I had a strong mindset that I wanted to be stronger through all the different martial arts out there. Rather than focusing on school education, I focused myself and my career in the path in creating teaching materials for the martial arts. Even though I knew I may not be able to make much money at the end, I wanted to follow my heart and my passion in the martial arts. Growing up, more than anything, I hated losing in any kind of a sport. Therefore, I exercised harder than anyone else. I always overly used my muscles, which forced me to carry around injury after injury. All the martial artists may look strong from the outside, but in comparison to everyday people, martial artists on the inside, they are the number one people that carry around all different kinds of chronic diseases. Around that time frame, I was entirely focused on pursuing myself to live a healthy lifestyle and that's when I met a colleague of mine who introduced me to "Sundo." During this time, Meditation, Zen, and Qigong community were very popular. In my short mindset youth, "Ki" caught my interest and it's mysteriousness behind it was mind boggling. I was hesitant in pursuing this path because of the people that surrounded me. Everyday people and the aged. That's when my colleague's parents were suffering from high blood pressure and diabetes, and through participating in "Sundo" practice, they were fully cured. That's when I questioned myself, is it really possible to cure these chronic illnesses and the incurable diseases through "Sundo" practice without having to visit the hospital? That motived me to take a closer look at the practice. In my very first "Sundo" practice,

I had to do 40 minutes of breathing practice, which is the key practice in "Sundo." After, I felt my body lighten up and gain more energy and strength. At that time, I thought weight training was the only way to develop strength. However, in doing the breathing exercises I was surprised and thrilled to see myself gain power and energy. Then, I finally realized this is what I've been looking for and I made a pledge to myself that I would continue with this all my life. I've been called teacher/coach/master in other sports and martial arts, but for "Sundo", in my second class, with a white belt around my waist, I made a promise to myself to give my full passion in practicing this art. Even to this very day, I don't believe that I am someone's master, rather I want to continue spreading my learnings and passion for this art with everyone that I meet because I also am still in the training process and will always keep on learning this art. I believe that having passion and wanting to do something in life is something we all need to be thankful for. If I could further expand my thoughts for "Sundo" and why I published this book, there are different books out there for this art in Korean, but it's regretful to see that their isn't one for English, which is the universal language in the world. That is the main reason why I went ahead to published this book. I want this book to be beneficial to this world and help those who are in need through "Sundo" practice.

II. BEFORE GETTING TO THE MAIN CONTENTS

Sundo have been passed on under various different names in the mountains for thousands of years, for examples, Bakdolbup, Kouksundo, Poongryudo, Goshindo etc. In 1967, the grandmaster cheongsan ,descended from the mountains in accordance with the orders of his master, began to announce in Korean society. At that time, Korean society was difficult economically and social awareness was not interested in Sundo practicing. Nevertheless, he tried to spread out with his sincere heart and soul. He showed a lot of demonstrations beyond human abilities to announce the Sundo.

He went back to mountain in 1985, and Currently, it has become a representative internal practice group in Korean society, has been maintaining legitimacy by his student who are faithful and sincere.

Here I'm saying that I have been written to fit modern and English expression based on his books and materials. I would like to express my gratitude the grandmaster Cheongsan and I want to able to reveal a little bit to the world which is infinite practice. Lastly I hope to see more advanced English version book regarding Sundo in the

future generation.

Modern people getting weak physically and getting bad emotionally. So, as a way to solve this social phenomenon,

I'm introducing the traditional Korean practice 'Sundo'.

III. Origin of Sundo

The ancient Korean ancestors worshiped the sun and performed a lot of ceremonies in which the people and the universe were united. In a practical way, they went up to the mountain to the closest sky and stretched the body evenly, stabilized the mind and controlled their breathing. Gradually, the practice has been systematized and historically developed. In short, people receive the brightness of the sun in the sky and actively participate in the universe change rule that turns around.

IV. Philosophy of Sundo

Sundo is a way that anyone can practice beyond religion, border, philosophy, and ideology, and also its fundamental thought is to view the universe, human being or nature, and human beings as one. We call this idea 'Gaejeonilyeogwan'. In other words, Everything under the sky will be seen as one. Since we are a part of nature, we must be assimilated into the laws and rules of nature to live in accord with the heavens. In that way, I suggest the Danjeon breathing in the Sundo practice.

In addition, Sudo aims to make the Hongikingan, that is, all living things on earth, to be widely benefited. In order to achieve this goal, we must cultivate extreme physical strength, extreme mental strength and noble sense of morality through self-training from myself. Ultimately aiming to become a holistic human being, and to help other people based on their vitality.

V. WHY IS SUNDO NECESSARY FOR MODERN PEOPLE?

If we summarize the ills of modern society in one word, we can say that the body becomes weak and the mind becomes bad. As a result of advanced material civilization, people are suffering from stress-related neurological diseases due to lack of proper exercise and mental labor occupy a relatively dominant position. We are also seeing that illness develops one step ahead as medicines and medicine develop. Numerous people are worried about what can fundamentally heal and resolve such illnesses.

In Sundo practicing, it is the position to borrow the power of the mother nature to be able to cure such social ills and we can get a solution by looking at the living philosophical principles of the Korean ancestors. It is said to be breathing. People often say that breathing exercises are daily even if they do not exercise. A few people know that there is a hidden secret in breathing to strengthening the body and mind. What we need to keep out health is earth energy(food), water and air. We can maintain life without eating a month, but breathing is enough to have a life-threatening effect even if we hold it for two minutes, and we cannot live for a while without breathing. Nowadays, in mass media, there are a lot of focus on food, such as what foods are nutritious, people should have vegetable and organic, which should be eaten according to what constitution, and in the information flood era, many people are rather wandering. We must realize that the kind and condition of food we eat with a mouth is important, and that the way in which what attitude, or in what way we breathe, has a profound effect on our bodies and minds. Grandmaster Cheongsan said the most common is the most healthful. I am convinced that we can heal the body and mind sickness if we intake proper seasonal food and acquire the breathing method.

VI. WHAT IS THE DANJEON OR DOLDANJARI?

It is said 'Jung'(essence) that the energy of the sky and the energy of the earth meet and gather. The energy of the sky is the energy from the air, and the energy of the earth is the energy from the grain and water. Jung which is gathered with these two energy are revealed by the power of the essence that can be seen and the power of the invisible spirit. These two things work together to move together as you think and decide. Therefore, Jung can be the root of the human body. There is a place where Jung is gathered by relying on both kidneys, it is egg-sized and fog or dew like intangible organs are danjeon. This important Jung is gathered in danjeon and continues to send to the whole body again and Jung is considered to be a treasure house which is the source of power. Danjeon is divided into upper, middle, and lower, and usually refers to the lower one (Hadanjeon). If the energy of the lower danjeon is strong, the energy of the upper and middle one are also clear and bright. It is same principle that the tree should have strong roots for getting healthy leaves and stems. For one more example, if the candle is big, the flame is strong and the light is bright and wide. So, it is most important to strengthen the low danjeon.

VII. Principle of Sundo

The mind is a vessel of thought, and the body is a vessel of mind. In the end, we practice mind through the body, Sundo emphasizes the moral fulfill by taking the power of practice based on the fullness of life through danjeon breathing. Sundo emphasizes deep breathing to obtain such strong vitality and noble character. As we live, we live without knowing the gratitude of breathing. If you look at breathing well, your mind is rough and emotional, your breathing becomes rough and shortened. On the other hand, when the breathing becomes longer and deeper, the mind becomes calm, peaceful, and able to think and act properly in every affair. If you want to breathe deeply, you will concentrate your mind on your lower abdomen and concentrate your mind. By concentrating your consciousness, energy can be collected and your body's energy source can be full. Breathing comes in and out through the low abdomen, the cerebral cortex, which has been excited in daily life, can be rested and the midbrain and the diencephalon that are responsible for our life support and natural healing powers get revitalized, the natural healing power is strengthened and can be recovered from most of diseases. In addition, the harmonization of autonomic nerves and strengthening of the abdominal pressure strengthens the digestion and absorption function, the excretory function going smoothly, the flow of blood in the liver and kidney is increased, and all the toxins of our body are filtered and decomposed, It is possible to maintain the health of the whole body, such as maintaining blood and energy and enhancing reproductive function as well. Moreover, when the breathing becomes longer, the breathing deepens naturally and then the thought wave goes down. And then you will be created the psychological relaxation in all the things and you will get the solemn character too.

People are looking for reasons to get sick from genetic, eating, hygienic, and psychological things. However, the biggest reason in Sundo is that when the harmony of mind and breathing is broken, the stable structure of energy becomes inverted pyramid from pyramid. So, the lower body becomes poor, the upper body becomes hardened, and diseases are appeared such as frozen shoulder, neck disc, migraine etc. Our body is called microcosm. The most ideal body state is that the upper body above the navel resembles the sky character which is always light and empty and the lower body is similar to the character of the earth like firm and hard. Therefore, if you practice danjeon breathing, you can feel that the energy is stable naturally, the lower body becomes stronger and the upper body becomes lighter. Also, when we sleep, adults are breathing deep into the belly while one is unconscious, so the tiredness is released after sleeping. In the end, concentrating on the danjeon intentionally in the training of the Sundo and breathing deeply at a steady speed make the immunity of our body increases naturally, the natural healing power is made. So, the illness of the body, mind disappears by itself and the mind also becomes calm and peaceful. Therefore, we get less stimulated from external stress and can be free from such stress. I would like to say that Sundo practice is not an unreliable or irrational but a rational and commonsensical practice. I think that truth is ordinary and should be understandable and acceptable for everyone. There is no expediency or a shortcut in Sundo practice. And it is not acquiring knowledge, knowing it as a head, but emphasizing practice with body and it is important to practice to get wisdom and ability by training yourself. Before you start practicing, you should practice emptying thoughts first. It does not make any sense to fill in something else while the desk drawer is full. In order to practice well, you should concede your own thoughts, stubbornness, and a little knowledge. And you should get attitude to accept the energy of the sky with humility in front of the nature, and communicate with the nature. Also, the result can be different depending on how much you devote to sincere breathing. In order to accomplish the each goal, we should do as if the cow plows the field simply and honestly.

VIII. BREATHING & LIFE

People are looking for reasons to get sick from genetic, eating, hygienic, and psychological things. However, the biggest reason in Sundo is that when the harmony of mind and breathing is broken, the stable structure of energy becomes inverted pyramid from pyramid. So, the lower body becomes poor, the upper body becomes hardened, and diseases are appeared such as frozen shoulder, neck disc, migraine etc. Our body is called microcosm. The most ideal body state is that the upper body above the navel resembles the sky character which is always light and empty and the lower body is similar to the character of the earth like firm and hard. Therefore, if you practice danjeon breathing, you can feel that the energy is stable naturally, the lower body becomes stronger and the upper body becomes lighter. Also, when we sleep, adults are breathing deep into the belly while one is unconscious, so the tiredness is released after sleeping. In the end, concentrating on the danjeon intentionally in the training of the Sundo and breathing deeply at a steady speed make the immunity of our body increases naturally, the natural healing power is made. So, the illness of the body, mind disappears by itself and the mind also becomes calm and peaceful. Therefore, we get less stimulated from external stress and can be free from such stress.

I would like to say that a Sundo practice is not an unreliable or irrational but a rational and commonsensical practice. I think that truth is ordinary and should be understandable and acceptable for everyone. There is no expediency or a shortcut in Sundo practice. And it is not acquiring knowledge, knowing it as a head, but emphasizing practice with body and it is important to practice to get wisdom and ability by training yourself.

Before you start practicing, you should practice emptying thoughts first. It does not make any sense to fill in something else while the desk drawer is full. In order to practice well, you should concede your own thoughts, stubbornness, and a little knowledge. And you should get attitude to accept the energy of the sky with humility in front of the nature, and communicate with the nature. Also, the result can be different depending on how much you devote to sincere breathing. In order to accomplish the each goal, we should do as if the cow plows the field simply and honestly.

Let's briefly describe the relationship between breathing methods and lifespan of animals. Turtles breathe 2-3 times a minute, their lifetime is 250-300 years, an elephant breathing 5-6 times a minute, lifetime is 150-200 years, and a person breathing 20-25 times per minute, The life span is 70 ~ 80 years and the dog breaths 80 ~ 90 times per minute. The life span is 15 ~ 25 years. We can see that respiration and lifespan are directly related. The main movement of the involuntary muscle and the voluntary muscle which is the diaphragm, allows us to take a deep breath that we desire. Let's look at what happens in our bodies when we breathe deeply.

In normal adults, the width of up and down movement of the diaphragm due to the usual breathing is about 2cm, and the circulation amount of air comes in and out about 0.5 liters (500cc). By the way, when you do danjeon breathing, the width of the diaphragm moves up to 6cm ~ 8cm, and the diaphragm goes down by 1cm. Also, the amount of air is increased about 0.25 liters (250cc) and so we can inhale 1.5 ~ 2 liters (1500 ~ 2000cc)) that we always supply the necessary oxygen in every part of our body. Thus, if you are a white-collar worker or a student who needs constant mind concentration, you can get good effect with clear mind without getting tired. Danjeon breathing also burns unnecessary fat in the body with a supply of oxygen, which is very helpful for healing adult diseases such as obesity, high blood pressure, diabetes and fatty liver. And the branches of the autonomic nerves that descend from the diencephalon through the active movement of the diaphragm are connected to the spine of the diaphragm to give good stimulation so that the natural healing power of the midbrain and diencephalon is activated. Moreover, helping the tension and relaxation action of the organs with stable deep breathing make the sympathetic nerve and the parasympathetic nerve are harmonized, so the autonomic nerves are regulated and strengthened.

In addition, there are trillions of cells in the human body. 10% of the cells divide daily and produce new cells. When the cell divides, the DNA is also divided in half, and here comes the reason for deep breathing. During cell division, the DNA in the nucleus is divided in half, and the DNA of the original information is copied. When you want to be able to copy the DNA correctly, you have to be in a healthy state to make the division without any mistake. When the best time for cell division is sleeping or relaxation is enough. If a person continues to undergo cell division despite being stressed and injured, DNA damage will occur. When the cell divides, misinformation is transmitted, mutation occurs, and disease occurs. Especially in the case of cancer, it is caused by DNA damage. So deep breathing in a calm state is a necessary thing for us, and we should see it as a necessity, not an option.

IX. ENTRANCE OF BREATHING PRACTICE

Before starting the danjeon breath, we do inner observation first in Sundo. Consciousness and breathing are closely related to each other like a coin's back and front. If the mind is not stable, rough, breathing is also rough, irregular. So ahead of a full-scale practice, let's concentrate your consciousness between eyebrows. Stay there about 5 seconds to look inside your body and look down at the nose. And slowly come down and look at your mouth quietly. And slowly look at your neck as observe your body. Then, while looking at the chest, consciousness gradually comes down to the belly. Then you look into your belly button and below the belly button. You can imagine that there is a big ball in there and you think there is nothing above the navel. This idea is not only to learn the basics, but always thinks that even when the stage goes up. You think there is no navel up, observing the belly quietly. If you look calmly at your belly, you can feel calm and relaxed, and when you are calm, your breathing can deepen and get longer. Although breathing techniques are important, you need to be aware that mindfulness in practicing is more important.

It is always good to have a humble, comfortable attitude in front of Mother Nature, as if you are in the arms of your mother. If you are a person of religion, you need to have a sense of embracing everything with the sense of being in the arms of Jesus or Buddha etc. Just as this earth, where we stand, have the rich and the poor, jewels, and dirt, and it is all without any discrimination, the mind of the practitioner should also have that kind of mind that can be helped in well-practicing. You need to open your mind, and accepts everything with all the sadness, joy and anger with a calm attitude. Keeping your mind closed and breathing is like breathing with the pathway of breathing blocked. Practicing means to manage your mind and boost up your vitality. It is not only training the body, but also control mind.

After the preparatory exercise is over, lay down comfortably with opened legs. Relax the tension of the abdominal muscles, and put both hands together and the thumb goes over the navel and gradually inhale through the nose with focusing on beneath the navel. When you breathe in, you feel that the bottom of your low abdomen is swollen up. It seems to stop for a while. When I breathe out, you feel that the belly returns to its original position. After exhale, you breathe like this repeatedly and naturally. At this time, take a breath in and out with adjusting almost the same. At the beginning, you can practice 5 sec in and 5 sec out. The length of the breathing should extend little by little naturally.

Do not give too much force at this time. Stiffen and blunt diaphragm muscles should be gently restored with the breathing. If it becomes habit to force the abdomen, In particular, it can be stifling as feels like pain in the chest due to the contraction of the diaphragm. It is very important to breathe according to your body condition and state of mental concentration. You can try to breathe in various postures.

For examples, put your hands on your low abdomen, try your arms wide open, face down with gathering your feet, place your cheeks on left or right, put your arms on your sides, sit or stand. Once you have become accustomed to breathing in various postures, you will be instructed by your instructor to begin the first stage of Sundo, which is Joonggidanbup former.

Warmup Exercise

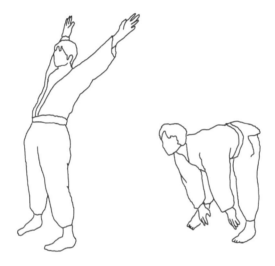

1. In shoulder length apart, place your two feet firmly on the ground to stretch our your whole body. Now breath in. While you breath in, stretch out both of your arms in the air and feel the energy at your fingertips and at the tip of your toes. This exercise puts the body in the manner of thanking the sky and the earth below us. Effectiveness includes relief of stress, stifling sensation in the chest, shoulder pain and relaxed body and mind

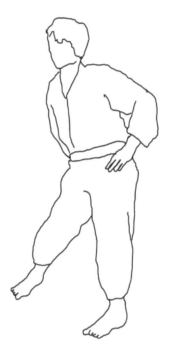

2. Surround the back of your waist, where the kidney's are with the palm of your hand and make a circular movement. Moving left and right three times. As you proceed on with this movement, make sure the circles get wider and wider each time. Effectiveness include relief of constipation and lower back pain.

3. Slowly sit down and place your two feet together and straighten out your two legs forward. Using all your fingertips, press firmly onto the ground. If you do not wish to use your fingertips, you can go ahead and use the palm of your hand. Now straighten out your spine and neck and open up your chest. Move your ankle forward and backwards four times and in circular motion, move your ankle left and right four times. Make sure to not bend your knees and send all of your strength/energy to your fingertips to keep balance. Effectiveness include dyspepsia, stomach disorder, headache, calf edema.

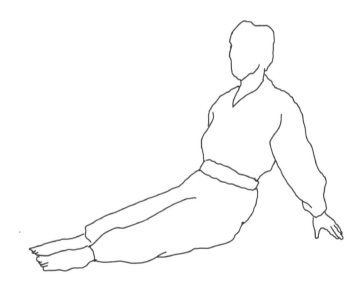

4. Now relax your mind and soul. By using the palm of your hand, start tapping from the tip of your toes to your lower stomach. Alternate your hands to tap around the different parts of your body. Shoulders, arms, wrist, again from your chest to stomach, onto your waist. This exercise helps with sending energy to different areas of your body and helps with blood circulation.

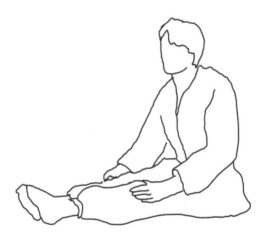

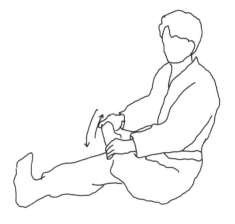

5.   Straighten out your right leg forward, and bend your
left leg and place your left knee over the right knee. Take
your left hand and place it over the left ankle and take your
right hand and place it on your left instep. Now take a deep
breath. While holding your breath, send Ki(Qi) energy
all the way to your fingertips and push and pull your body
for about four times. You may move from your ankle and
below, but by using your left hand, hold on to your ankle
so that it doesn't move from ankle and above. Now breathe
out and breathe in again. While holding your breath, move
your ankle in both directions four times in a circular motion
and then breathe out. For the people who can't breathe for
a long time, do not force long breathing exercises onto the
body. It may cause the Ki(Qi) energy to go in the opposite
direction. Make sure to find your own breathing pattern
that suit your body. This exercise prevents ankle disease, loss
of appetite, astrodynamics.

6. In the same position as number 5, now place your right hand over your left ankle. After, make a fist with your left hand and tap the left sole of your feet 10 times. Then by using your thumb press firmly once again into your sole. This exercise prevents paralysis of both legs, hypertension, cystitis, and nerve disease.

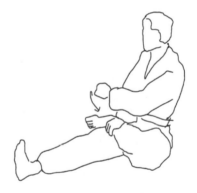

7. In the same position as number 5, start gathering all your fingers from your index finger to your pinky. Then, in using your pinky, cover the half of your malleolus and use your right thumb and place it right below the bones and fold your left thumb. Now breathe in. Hold your breath and straighten your waist and arms and press gently into the area. This is an acupuncture point, where meridian intersects between Kidney, Liver, and Spleen. This benefits while stimulating these three viscera areas. This prevents irregular menstruation, period pain, low abdomen pain, indigestion contraindication. Women who are pregnant, it is not ideal and preferred not press into this area.

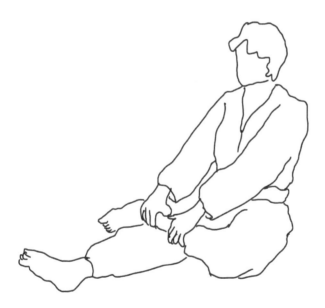

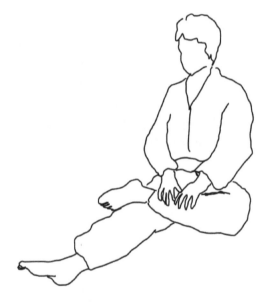

8. In the same position, lightly press inwards to your calf muscles surrounding the tibia area and thighs. This prevents paralysis of both legs, and urethritis.

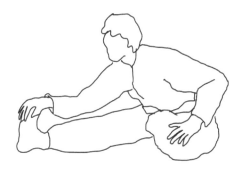

9. In the same position, place your left ankle over your right knee. Take your right hand and hold onto your toes or your ankle. With your left hand hold onto your left knee and gently press down. In using your upper body, lean forward then lean forward 45 degrees and then lean deeply more forward. This realigns the spine, and prevents coxitis, pelvic inflammatory disease, irregular menstruation, and indigestion.

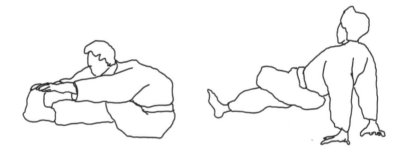

10. In the same position, straighten your spine starting from the hypogastric region. Lean forward towards your feet and hold onto your toes or ankle. Now swing left and right. Then, take both of your hands, and place it behind you in using your fingers or the palm of your hand. Slowly push your body up and swing left and right. Then, center your body to the hypogastric region, and push your body further up and then come back down to your original position. Repeat this exercise two times. This prevents indigestion and strengthens abdomen.

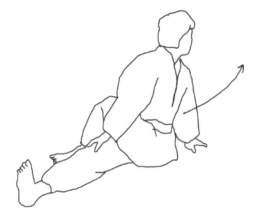

11. In the same position, raise your left knee and place it on the outer edge of the right knee. Then, shadowing your right hand, place your elbow on the outer edge of the left knee and hold your right knee area, (If this positions causes discomfort, you may take your right hand and place it over the outer are of your left knee and hold). Now raise your left fingers and place it behind your tail bone. Now breathe in. While holding your breath, slowly start turning from your tail bone to each joint in your spine to your neck bone. Then while breathing out, slowly turn back to your original position starting with your neck bone to your tail bone. Repeat this exercise two times. This prevents lower back pain, shoulder pain and helps with slimming your waist and correcting the pelvis.

12. Repeat number 5 with the opposite side.
13. Repeat number 6 with the opposite side.
14. Repeat number 7 with the opposite side.
15. Repeat number 8 with the opposite side.
16. Repeat number 9 with the opposite side.
17. Repeat number 10 with the opposite side.
18. Repeat number 11 with the opposite side.

19. Now open up your feet wide to left and right. Then, press softly near the thigh area and tap lightly. (Don't forget to always give tension at the tip of your toes). With your feet staying in the same position, now breathe in. While holding your breath, twist your upper body and place your left fingers behind your tail bone and your right fingers lightly touching the ground. Now start bending your left elbow and lean your upper body backwards giving pressure. Then, in breathing out, start unwinding your body. Now do this same exercise with the right side. Repeat two times. This prevents sciatica, hernia, irregular menstruation, and strengthens pelvic, ovary stimulation.

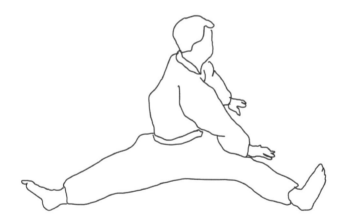

20. In the same position, gather your both hand into the hypogastric region. In raising your both hands, straighten your spine and lean towards your left holding onto your toes or ankle. Now swing left and right. Do the same thing for the right side. Repeat two times. This strengthens brachialis muscle, abdominal muscle, finger bone and sinews, vertebra, cervical area, and prevents myopia.

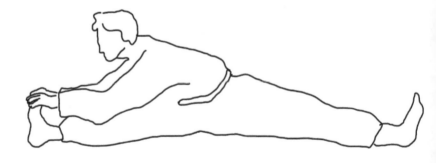

21. In the same position, straighten your waist and slowly bend your upper body forward. (At this time, the main focus, hypogastric area, is touching the ground and bend forward as much as you can. All these positions may cause difficulty at first, but in training your body with the breathing exercises these positions will come naturally without force and discomfort).

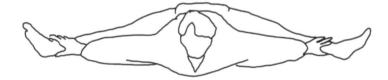

22. In the same position, raise up your upper body and place both of your hands behind your back. Hold firmly onto the ground, using your fingers. Raise your body and twist left and right. Then, raise up your hypogastric region up to the sky and come back to position. This exercise helps with indigestion, stifling sensation in the chest, and leg muscle pain. Repeat number 21 and 22 two times each.

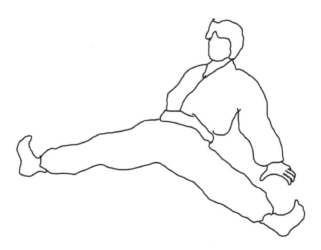

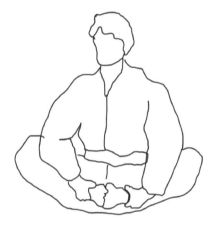

23. Now place the sole of your left and right foot together. Take your both hand and place them onto both of your knees. Gently press down and release. Repeat three times. This prevents constipation, prostate, menstrual pain, cystitis, incongruity hip joint and helps with reproductive system.

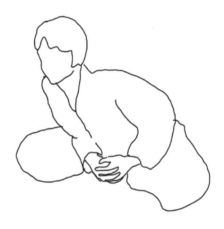

24. Take both of your hands and hold onto each ankle. Having the outer edge of your feet touching the ground, hold up your body up and down. Repeat three times. This prevents sciatica, menstrual pain, and strengthens ankle.

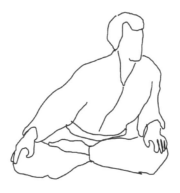

25. Take both of your hands and cover your toes and firmly pull inwards. Then lean your upper body forward and up. Then, taking only the orientation of your face, turn left and bend down and up, then turn right and bend down and up. This prevents hernia, testicle pain, irregular menstruation, and sciatica.

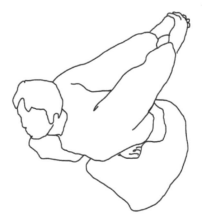

26. Take full cross position, group - (Bend your right leg and place it in the inner edge of your left thigh. Bend your left leg and come inward towards the right leg and fold over. At this point, if full cross position doesn't work, just take one leg and place it over the opposite thigh). Now place both of your hand over the knee and straighten your spine and fully open up your chest. Then, in a big circular motion, move your upper body left and right three times each. This prevents lower back pain, leukorrhea, stifling sensation in the chest.

27. In the full cross position, place both of your hands behind your back and lock your fingers together. Twist your upper body to the left and bend down and up, do the same on your right side. Repeat two times. Turn back to the center of your attention and bend over forward and up and then take your locked fingers and swing your arm left and right. Repeat two times. This prevents intercostal neuralgia, chest pain, cold, lung disease, constipation and promotes digestive power.

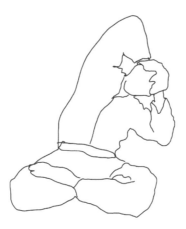

28. In the full cross position, place both of your hands behind your neck and lock your fingers together. Bend your upper body towards the left then to the right. When you are bending over to each side, make sure the opposite side of your body is fully stretched. Repeat two times. This prevents scoliosis and astrodynamics.

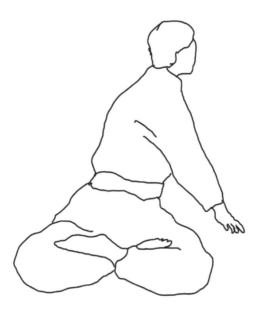

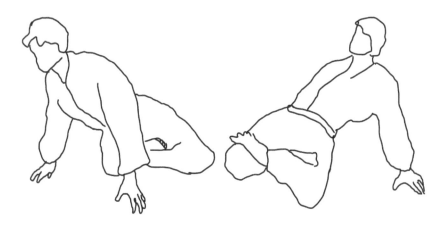

29. In the full cross position, twist your upper body toward the left while placing your left fingers on the tail bone. Bend your left elbow while your right fingers touch the ground. Now bend backwards. Do the same for your right side and repeat two times. This prevents lower back pain and lower abdomen pain.

30. In the full cross position, start moving up your upper body and start to stand on your knees. While following your upper body and your knees, use all your fingers to support and step far forward. Pull your head in the forward motion and twist left and right. (At this point, in while following your upper body, have your chest area touch the ground and push forward. While pulling back up, have your hypogastric region reach the ground in a rhythmical motion). Then, pull your upper body backwards, using all your fingertips to hold onto the ground and having the hypogastric region become the center of your energy raise up your body up and down. Repeat two times. This strengthens vertebra, costal and prevents stomach disorder.

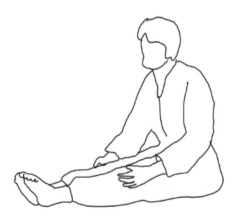

31. Now release your legs from the full cross position and straighten out your legs forward and shake out your legs by using your feet. Use both of your hands to tap and loosen the tension starting from the tip of your toes to the inner and outer areas of your legs. Alternating between the hand tap around your shoulders, arms and the hypogastric region.

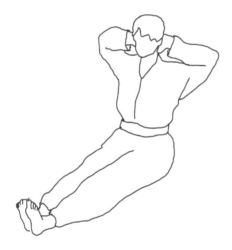

32. Straighten out both of your legs and raise up the tip of your toes. In this position, straighten up your spine and place both of your hands behind your neck and lock your fingers together. Now lean forward and pull back up. Straighten your waist then twist your upper body to the left. Again, lean forward and pull back up, then twist to the right. Repeat two times. This prevents gastroenteric trouble, common cold, and helps fatigue recovery and low blood pressure.

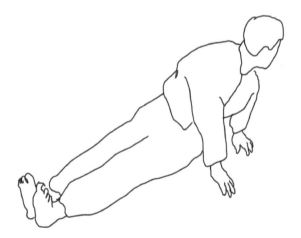

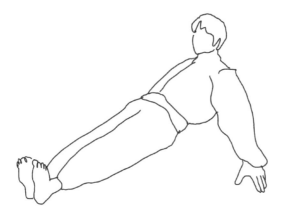

33. In the same position, twist your upper body to the left and place your left fingers on your tail bone. Then, bend your left elbow and have your right fingers touch the ground. Now lean backwards to the maximum. Do the same thing on your right side. Repeat two times. This prevents lower back pain and irregular menstruation.

34. Straighten out your body, then, in facing each other, place both of your hand in the hypogastric region. Raise up your arms while straightening out your spine and lean forward. Now hold onto your toes or your ankle and swing left and right. Then, take all your fingers and place it behind you. In holding onto the floor with all your fingers, push your body upward and twist left and right, making sure the hypogastric region is reaching up to the sky at it's maximum. Repeat two times. This helps with digestive disorder, constipation, nasal congestion, lower back pain, abdomen, waist, slimmer legs and takes off surplus fat.

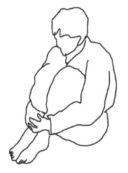
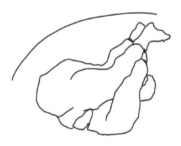

35. Gather your feet together and bend your knees upward. Lock your fingers together and cover over the lower regions of your knees. Then, push your upper body backwards and roll back and forth 10 times. This helps spine manipulation, lower back pain, insomnia, vitality recovery.

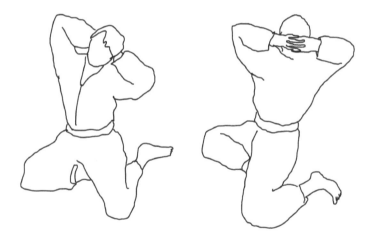

36. Bend both of your knees and have only your left leg face outward. Place both of your hands behind your neck and lock your fingers together. Then, have your upper body fall to the left and back up. Then, straighten out your arms and your upper body and twist to the right. Repeat two times. In the same position, just alternate between two legs and repeat the same exercise two times. This helps with shoulder pain, neck area blood circulation disorder, intercostal neuralgia, lower back pain.

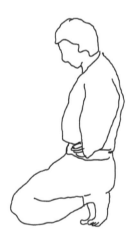

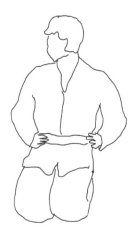

37. Raise up your toes and bend your knees. Take both of your hands and place it at the each side of your waist. Then, have your neck fall forward and backward. Repeat 8 times. This helps with cervical relaxation, respiratory system, shoulder pain, stiffness of the neck and shoulders.

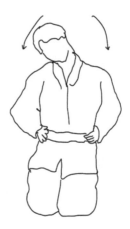

38. Turn your head to the left and to the right eight times.

39. In the image of having your ear fall to your shoulder, fall forward left and right eight times. At this times, not only are you releasing tension in your shoulders, you have to make sure the flank of opposite sides are fully straightened out.

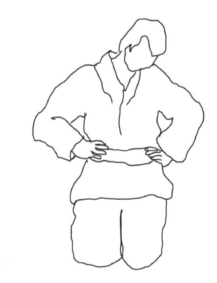

40. Now open your eye wide. In a circular motion, circle around left and right three times each.

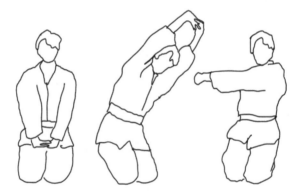

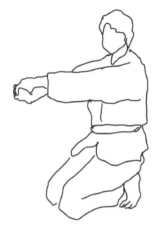 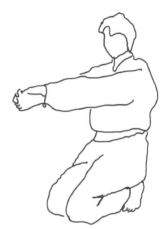

41. In the same position, lock your fingers together. Now fall to the bottom, then push forward and twist left and right. Again, with your fingers locked together, come towards your chest area and twist left and right. This helps with shoulder stiffness, strengthens cardiopulmonary function, and tinnitus. Especially, pushing outward with your locked fingers helps with hand/foot pain, rheumatism, nervous breakdown, anxiety fatigue, thyroid disease.

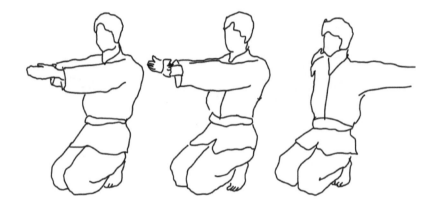

42. In the same position, lock your fingers together, but cross your fingers so that they are interlocking. Now draw towards your chest and circle back forward and straighten. Repeat two times, then, which hands and repeat two times again.

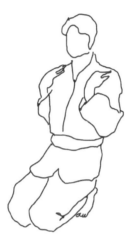

43. 1)Now have the palm of your hands face each other.
In putting pressure onto your fingertips, push forward and
lean widely to open up your chest to each side. Repeat three
times. 2)Now have the back of your hands face each other
and repeat exercise 1 (above) three times. 3)Now have the
thumbs face each other and repeat exercise 1 (above) three
times. 4)Now have your pinkies face each other and repeat
exercise 1 (above) three times. In doing these exercises,
it is very important that you remember to put pressure
at your fingertips and push forward. The first exercise
should be done slowly, but it is important to remember, in
pushing forward, to make sure you receive the feeling of
your shoulder blades touching each other. This helps with
stifling sensation in your chest, bronchitis, shoulder pain,
strengthen cardiopulmonary function.

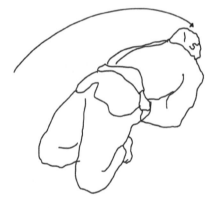

44. Place both of your on each shoulder. In a wide circular motion, lean forwards three and backwards three times. This helps with paralysis and arm spasm.

45. Straighten out our waist. Then, support both of your hands on your waist. Slowly lean backwards. At this point, it is important to have elasticity in your whole body. In having the center of your weight fall below, have your head naturally fall through together. This helps strengthen cardiopulmonary, activation of digestive system, bronchitis, spine manipulation, and balance of the pelvis.

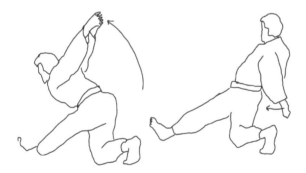

46. In your kneeling position, place our your left foot 45 degrees. Then, place both of your hands behind you, and in facing your palms, lock your fingers together. Now lower your upper body towards your left foot, and come back up, and swing left and right. At this point, when your are lowering your body, make sure your chin faces far outwards. Repeat to the left/right two times. This helps with shoulder stiffness, indigestion, abdomen pain, and knee pain.

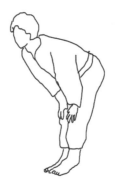

47. Now slowly stand up. Place each of your hands on your knees and alternate between sitting down and standing up. Repeat three times. At this point, make sure the heels of your feet are firmly pressed down onto the floor. This helps with knee pain.

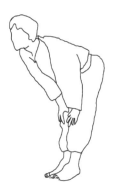

48. In the same position, hold onto your knees and circle widely around to your left and right three times. This helps with knee pain and sciatica.

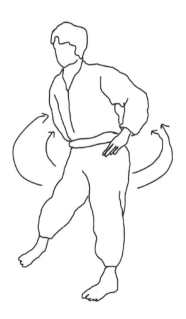

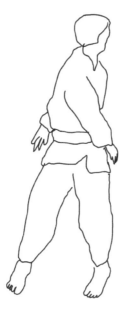

49. In your standing up position, place your hands on your waist and circle widely around to your left and right three times. This helps with lower back pain, constipation, strengthening of the organ functions.

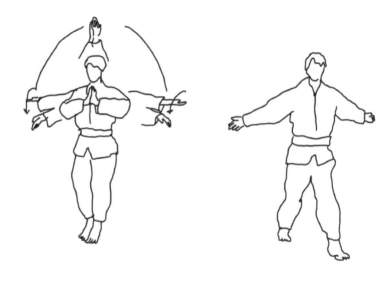

50. Now release all the tension in your body. After you fully relax your arms, put pressure in your hypogastric area and twist your arms to the left and to the right. This helps with whole body relaxation, gastroenteric trouble, balances the body, and gives flexible waist.

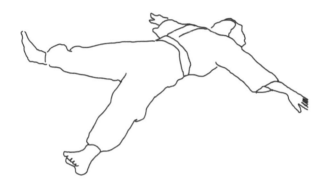

51. Gather your feet together. While you push up the heels of your feet, breath in and raise both of your hands upwards. Then, in a parallel motion, release it to the side. Now breathe out. Then while pushing your feet outward to 45 degrees, open your hands widely to left and right and breathe in. Then, while gathering your hands back inwards, breathe out. In breathing in, have the opposite foot go out and when the foot comes back in, breathe out. Do this for two times then rub your hands against each other to develop heat. Then, put it over your stomach and massage in circular motion. This helps with fatigue recovery, promotes metabolism, and improves blood circulation.

52. Now peacefully lay down and get ready to go into training. While you are laying down, open up your hands and feet to the comfort of your body and start breathing to stabilize your body and mind. This helps relax your mind, rest brain waves, and sleep well.

Wrap-up Exercise

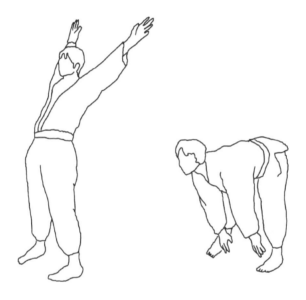

1. In the laid down position, think that you are sending the "Ki" energy to the very tip of your fingertips and to the very tip of your toes. Now using your arms and feet, stretch out your whole body. This exercise would be more beneficial, if you pull your spine up and down. This helps with gastroenteric trouble, abdomen pain, constipation, and arm pain.

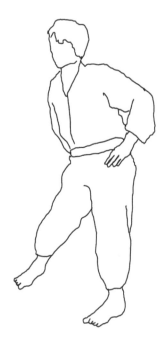

2. In the laid down position, straddle your feet to left and right. Place your hands behind your neck and lock your fingers together. Then twist left and right. This helps with shoulder pain, lower back pain, and prevents facial neuralgia.

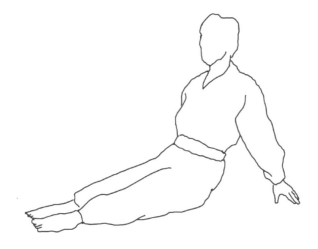

3. In the laid down position, rub your hands against each other to develop heat then rub against your face. Then, using the tip of your fingers, evenly press the eye and the cheekbone area. Next, evenly press the next of your nose, back of your neck, and your scalp. Then, hold onto your ears and pull them up and down giving stimulation. In giving stimulation to your face and head, it can stimulates your internal organs. This helps with headache, auditory difficulty and tinnitus.

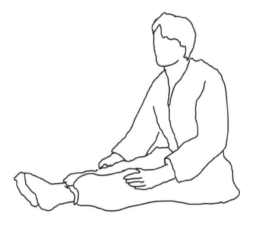

4. Hold onto your left shoulders with your right hand. In a circular motion, move your left arm starting from the back to the front three times, and in opposite direction three times. Do the same on your opposite arm. This helps with shoulder pain.

5. Stretch out both of your hands up and down six times. This helps with strengthening costal, flank pain, gastroenteric trouble.

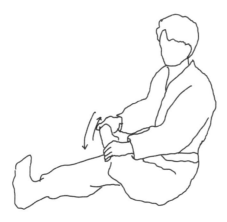

6. Make the motion of having your both arms hug around your chest, and stretch far out to your left and right. Repeat three times. This helps with shoulder pain, and strengthening the thyroid gland.

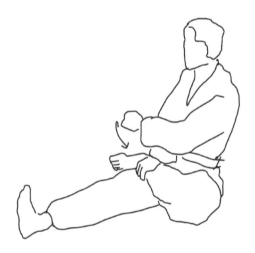

7. Raise both of your hands and feet and lightly shake them around.

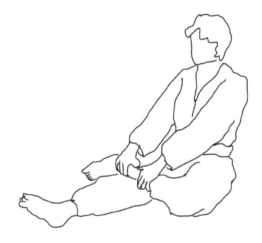

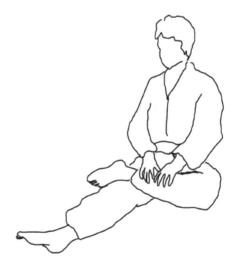

8. Place the palms of your hand on the floor and gather your feet together. Now bend your knees and twist to your left and right. At this point, make sure the direction of your face and the direction of your knees are opposite of each other. This way, you will feel the push and pull of the body. This helps with spine manipulation and lower back pain.

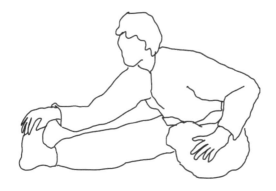

9. In the laid down position, place your hands on the floor. Gather your feet and raise them up to move them in a wide circular motion. Left two times and right two times. This helps with sciatica, food and leg spasm.

10. In the same position, raise up your left foot and with your left hand hold onto your knee. Hold your ankle with the right hand. In this position, bend your knees back and forth. Repeat three times. Do the same on the opposite side with alternate hands. Repeat three times. This helps with correcting pelvic osteotomy, and aid digestion.

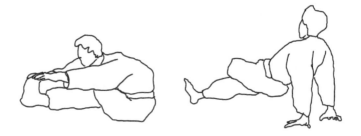

11. In the laid down position, place your hands on the floor and gather your feet together. Raise up the heels of your feet and place it right next to your hip. Then, hold up your whole body and twist to your left and right. When pulling back down, fully relax your body and stretch out your feet. Drop it to the ground, stimulating your body.

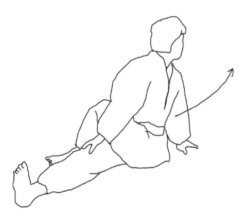

12. In the laid down position, gather your hands and feet. Now breathe in. Then, with your hip firmly grounded, slowly raise up your upper and lower body at the same time. Do not raise it up too high or drop it too low. Hold it up to the most moderate position to give enough tension to your hypogastric area and then release and relax.

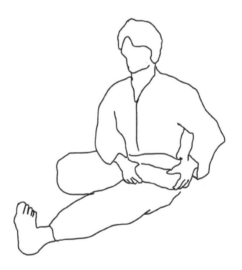

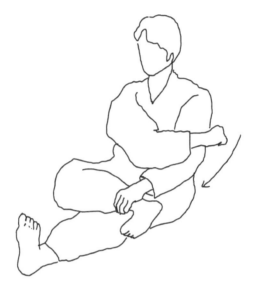

13. Open up your feet wide. Raise up your right hand and stretch out your left hand perpendicular to your side. Tilt your left hand and your upper body to the right. While having your chest touch the ground, send the hypogastric "Ki" energy to the tip of your finger tips. Do the same for the opposite side. This helps with headache, tonsillitis, and enhance costal.

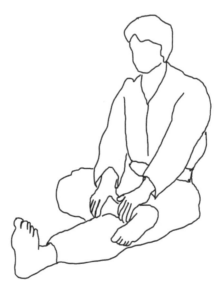

14. In the same position, place the palm of your hands on the ground and open up your hands and feet. Then, raise up your left foot and bring it over to where your right hand is located. Now twist your upper body to the left. Alternate and raise up your right foot and bring it over to where your left hand is located. Then, till your upper body to the right. This helps with lower back pain, spine manipulation, gastroenteric trouble.

15. In the laid down position, place your hands on your stomach. Gather your feet together. Now, by using your neck and the toes of your feet, slowly raise up your whole body and rock forward and backward stimulating your neck. At this point, gently close your mouth together. This helps with headache, tinnitus, eye disease, hemorrhoids, rhinitis, and sinus infection.

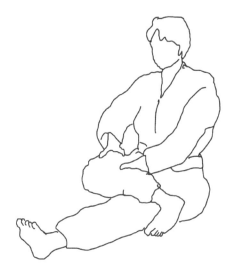

16. In the laid down position, gather your feet together and slowly flip it towards the back of your neck. With both of your hands, support your waist and bend your ankle back and forth, open up your feet far wide to your left and right, alternate from front and back, and cycle your legs as if you are riding a bicycle. In the end, slowly raise up your feet in perpendicular motion and send it over to the back of your head. Then, place both of your hands on the floor and slowly come back to the original position. This helps with splanchnoptosis, restore thyroid function, varicose vein, indigestion, constipation, spine manipulation, headache, neck and shoulder stiffness, rhinitis, nasal congestion, and sinus infection.

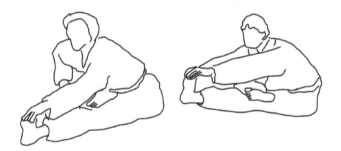

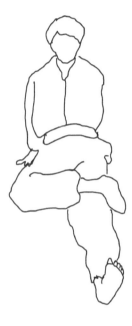

17. In the laid down position, place both of your hands in the shoulder area and gather your feet together. Then, bend your knees and place it on the floor. By using the strength of your toes and all your fingers, push up your whole body. If using your fingers give you discomfort, you may use the palm of your hands. Then, in the motion of lifting up your hypogastric area keep the tension throughout your whole body. This helps with depression, emotional stability, spine manipulation, constipation, renal calculi, cardiovascular activation.

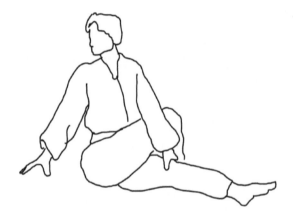

18. Slowly face downwards, and start knocking on the floor with your fingers and toes.

19. In the face down position, take both of your hands and place in the front of your shoulder. Now slowly start rising up. Starting with your head to your neck and then stimulating each joint of your spine. If possible, have your hypogastric region firmly on the ground. Slowly start twisting your upper body to your left and right. Then, move your head backwards and back to original position. This helps with better circulation of the intervertebral discs, cardiovascular activation, constipation, chronic diarrhea, indigestion, stomachache, and renal calculi.

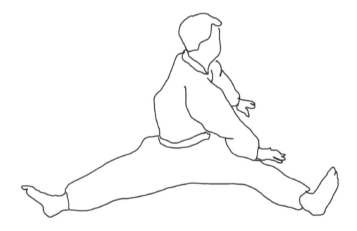

20. In the face down position, open up your feet. Stretch your right hand upwards and stretch your left hand to your side in the perpendicular motion. Slowly raise your left hand, then twist your upper body towards the right and then have the back of your hand touch the ground. Do the same for the opposite side. This helps with myasthenia gastrica, and actives kidney function.

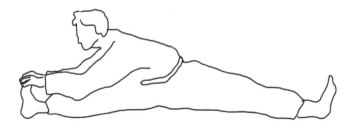

21. In the face down position, hold onto the ground with the palm of your hands and center your attention to the front. Raise the tip of your toes straight, then, gather your feet together. While the tip of your toes are still straight, slowly raise up your left foot to your maximum. Make sure the hypogastric region does not fall away from the floor. Also, your head, neck, and your spine has to be straight at all times. In contrary, now raise up your right leg. This helps with constipation, hemorrhoids, splanchnoptosis, lumber spine calibration, strengthens your kidney, and positions calibration of the uterus.

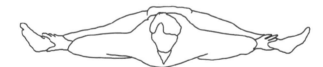

22. In the face down position, use your right hand to grab your left ankle and your left hand stretched outward to the front. Have part of your stomach touch the ground and raise up the rest your body upward. Now slowly rock your body back and forth. Alternate your hands and feet and do the same for the opposite side. This strengthens costal and spine and helps gastroenteric trouble.

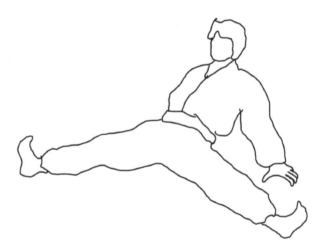

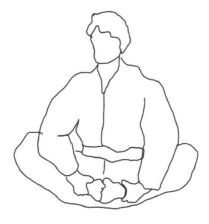

23. In only having the stomach area touch the ground, take both of your hands and grab onto each ankle. Now raise up your whole body and rock back and forth. This helps with light herniated disc, splanchnoptosis, irregular menstruation, uterine disease, obesity, removes extra fat from the liver of alcohol and promotes digestion.

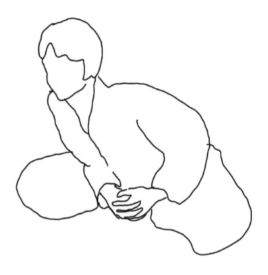

24. Place both of your hands on your waist and tap slowly, while your toes are knocking on the floor.

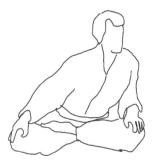

25. In the face down position, ground both of your hands and shoulders on the floor. Now kneel down then ground yourself to the floor as much as your can and push your upper body forward and up. Again, ground yourself to the floor as much as you can, and slowly start pushing out your hips in coming back to the original position. Then, start stimulating your body in the motion of pulling yourself to your left and right. Repeat three times to your right and left, then turn your body backwards to your maximum and come back to the original position. This helps with promotion of digestion, chronic diarrhea, constipation, uterine and urinary abnormality and cold constitution.

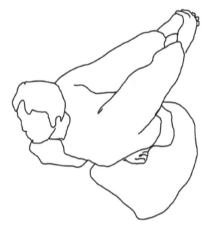

26. Now only place your fingers and your toes on the floor and raise up your whole body. In alternating your feet, start kicking upwards along with kicking up your lower body.

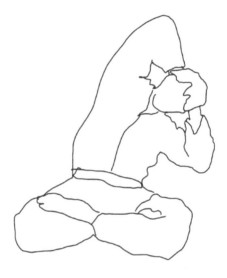

27. In releasing your body, lightly swing your body to your left and right and relax your whole body. Lightly and pleasantly, jump up and down in place. Then, lastly, start breathing. This helps with whole body energy circulation, releases stiffness, promotion of digestion, and prevents constipation.

Printed in Poland
by Amazon Fulfillment
Poland Sp. z o.o., Wrocław

33510235R10057